PREVENTING BLINDNESS

"Simple Steps to Protect Your Vision and Prevent Blindness"

By
Dr. Philip P. Longwell

Copyright

All rights reserved. No part of this publication may be reproduced, distributed, or transmitted in any form or by any means, including photocopying, recording, or other electronic or mechanical methods, without the prior written permission of the publisher, except in the case of brief quotations embodied in critical reviews and certain other noncommercial uses permitted by copyright law.

Copyright © Dr. Philip P. Longwell, 2023

Table of content

Introduction
Chapter 1
Chapter 2
Chapter 3
Chapter 4
Chapter 5
Conclusion
Recap of essential points

Introduction

Jack has always been captivated by the human body and its potential to repair itself. He had always been attracted to the medical industry, and he had spent years studying and researching different methods to cure various maladies.

One day, Jack came across a book that captivated his interest. It was named "Preventing blindness: "Simple Steps to Protect Your Vision and Prevent Blindness." Jack was fascinated by the title and soon started reading.

The book was full of information on the numerous eye disorders that might lead to blindness, as well as techniques to avoid and cure these problems. Jack was captivated by the different approaches and strategies that were detailed in the book, and he immediately became eager to put this information to use.

Over the following six months, Jack worked feverishly to learn as much as he could about eye health. He studied every book and paper he could find on the topic, and he even began volunteering at a local eye clinic to obtain hands-on experience.

As Jack continued to study, he came to grasp the need for frequent eye examinations and the role that diet and exercise had in keeping good eyesight. He also learned about the many treatments and surgeries that were available to address common eye problems such as cataracts and glaucoma.

Using the information he had received from the book, Jack was able to assist many individuals to avert blindness and keep the good vision. He was delighted to have discovered such a great resource, and he knew that he would continue to utilize it throughout his career in the medical industry.

Blindness is a severe affliction that may drastically damage a person's quality of life. It may lead to social isolation, difficulty with movement, and issues with everyday duties such as cooking and bathing. However, blindness is frequently avoidable. With adequate care and attention, it is possible to avert blindness and preserve excellent eye health. In this essay, we will cover several practical actions that may help you prevent blindness and keep your eyesight clear.

Chapter 1

What is blindness?

Blindness is the entire or partial inability to see, either due to a medical condition or damage. It may be caused by a multitude of circumstances, including heredity, illness, trauma, or other factors. People who are blind may not be able to see at all, or they may have some vision but not enough to accomplish routine chores without help. Blindness may be congenital, meaning it is present from birth, or it can develop later in life. Some frequent causes of blindness include glaucoma, cataracts, retinal detachment, and macular degeneration. Blindness may also be induced by injuries, such as those received in vehicle accidents or falls.

There are numerous varieties of blindness, including:

Complete blindness: This indicates that the individual is unable to see anything, including light or shadows.

Partial blindness: This indicates that the individual has some eyesight, but it is restricted. They may be able to see items that are close up or far away, but not both.

Low vision: This signifies that the individual has a vision that is considerably degraded, but not entirely gone. They may be able to see things and people but may have trouble with activities such as reading or driving.

Causes of blindness

There are various reasons for blindness, some of which include:

Inherited genetic problems: Some people may be born with genetic abnormalities that cause blindness, such as retinitis pigmentosa or albinism.

Cataracts: Cataracts are hazy patches in the lens of the eye that may hinder vision. They are frequent in elderly persons, but may sometimes arise in younger individuals owing to injury or continuous use of certain drugs.

Glaucoma: Glaucoma is a disorder that destroys the optic nerve, which sends visual information from the eye to the brain. It is generally caused by excessive pressure in the eye and may lead to blindness if left untreated.

Diabetic retinopathy: People with diabetes are at risk of developing diabetic retinopathy, a disorder that destroys the blood vessels in the retina. This may lead to visual loss or blindness.

Macular degeneration: Macular degeneration is a disorder that affects the center section of the retina, known as the macula. It may cause progressive eyesight loss and is frequent in elderly adults.

Damage or injury: Physical trauma to the eye or brain may cause vision loss or blindness.

Diseases: Certain infections, such as herpes simplex or chickenpox, may cause inflammation and damage to the eye and lead to vision loss.

Vitamin A shortage: A deficit in vitamin A may cause visual loss, particularly in children living in underdeveloped nations.

Age-related vision loss: As individuals age, their chance of having vision loss or blindness rises owing to disorders such as cataracts, glaucoma, and macular degeneration.

Importance of avoiding blindness

Blindness is an important public health concern that may have a considerable influence on an individual's quality of life. It may also lead to social isolation and a lack of independence, which can be emotionally and financially burdensome for the individual afflicted and their family.

Chapter 2

Preventing blindness is vital for various reasons:

It may increase the quality of life: Blindness can substantially impair an individual's ability to lead a normal life. It might make it difficult to conduct regular duties such as cooking, driving, or simply going for a stroll. By avoiding blindness, people may continue to enjoy their lives to the utmost.

It may lower the load on healthcare systems: Blindness can lead to a variety of additional health conditions, such as depression and anxiety, which can impose a major burden on healthcare systems. By avoiding blindness, we can lower the need for healthcare resources and free them up for other important needs.

It may save lives: In certain situations, blindness can lead to accidents or injuries, which can be deadly. By avoiding blindness, we can lower the likelihood of accidents and deaths.

It may help decrease poverty: Blindness can lead to lost income and a loss of independence, which can contribute to poverty. By avoiding blindness, we may help people preserve their livelihoods and alleviate poverty in the long run.

There are various strategies to prevent blindness, including frequent eye check-ups, wearing protective eyewear, eating a nutritious diet, and avoiding cigarettes and alcohol. By investing in preventive measures, we can assist guarantee that people preserve their sight and enjoy happy lives.

Maintaining excellent eye health is vital for protecting your eyesight and avoiding blindness. Here are some guidelines for keeping excellent eye health:

Get frequent eye exams: It is vital to get your eyes tested periodically, even if you don't have any visual difficulties. Eye examinations may uncover issues early on when they are most curable.

Wear protective eyewear: If you participate in activities that might hurt your eyes, such as playing sports or working with power tools, be sure to wear protective eyewear.

Protect your eyes from the sun: Excessive exposure to UV radiation may harm your eyes, therefore it is crucial to wear sunglasses that filter out UV rays while you are outside.

Eat a nutritious diet: A healthy diet that includes foods rich in vitamins A and C, as well as zinc and omega-3 fatty acids, will help maintain excellent eye health.

Don't smoke: Smoking is hazardous to your general health, and it may also raise your chance of developing eye disorders such as cataracts and age-related macular degeneration.

Take pauses from displays: Spending lengthy amounts of time gazing at devices may strain your eyes, thus it is necessary to take breaks and look away from the screen every 20 minutes.

By following these guidelines, you may assist maintain excellent eye health and lower your chance of having vision difficulties or going blind.

Chapter 3

Hand hygiene

Hand cleanliness is a key element in avoiding the transmission of sickness and disease, especially infections that may lead to blindness. There are various ways in which hand cleanliness might aid to lower the incidence of blindness:

Prevention of infections: Proper hand hygiene may assist to avoid the transfer of infectious organisms that can cause eye infections or other diseases that can lead to blindness. This involves washing hands routinely with soap and water, particularly after using the restroom or touching contaminated surfaces.

Avoiding eye injuries: Proper hand hygiene may also assist to limit the risk of eye injuries caused by filthy hands. For example, if you contact your eyes with filthy hands, you may accidentally scrape your eye or introduce germs or other impurities that might cause illness.

Reducing the transmission of sickness: Proper hand cleanliness may also assist to minimize the spread of illness to others. If you are unwell and have an eye infection or other condition that might lead to blindness, washing your hands often can assist to avoid the transfer of the sickness to others.

To practice appropriate hand hygiene, follow these steps:

1. Wet your hands with clean, running water (warm or cold) and apply soap.

2. Rub your hands together to generate a lather and scrub all areas, including the backs of your hands, and wrists, between your fingers, and beneath your nails.

3. Continue rubbing your hands for at least 20 seconds. Need a timer? Hum the "Happy Birthday" song from beginning to finish twice.

4. Rinse your hands thoroughly under clean, running water.

5. Dry your hands with a clean towel or air dry them.

By following these easy actions, you may help to lower the risk of blindness and other disorders associated with inadequate hand hygiene.

Proper usage of contact lenses

Proper usage of contact lenses is vitally crucial to prevent blindness. Contact lenses are a popular alternative for correcting eyesight, but they may potentially be harmful if not worn appropriately. Here are some ideas on how to correctly utilize contact lenses to prevent blindness:

Follow your doctor's directions: It is crucial to follow the instructions of your eye doctor when it comes to wearing and caring for your contact lenses. This covers how frequently to change them, how long to wear them each day, and how to clean and disinfect them.

Manage your lenses carefully: Contact lenses are sensitive, and it is necessary to handle them with care. Always wash your hands before handling your lenses, and avoid wearing them in circumstances where they might be easily damaged or misplaced.

Avoid wearing lenses for too long: It is necessary to take pauses from wearing contact lenses to enable your eyes to breathe. Wearing them for too long may lead to dry eyes, which can lead to vision difficulties.

Use the proper solution: It is crucial to use the correct solution to clean and disinfect your contact lenses. Using the improper solution might lead to discomfort and injury to the eyes.

Seek medical treatment if you suffer issues: If you experience any problems while using contact lenses, such as redness, irritation, or impaired vision, it is crucial to seek medical assistance as soon as possible. Ignoring these concerns might lead to major visual impairment and perhaps blindness.

By following these suggestions, you may guarantee that you are wearing your contact lenses safely and properly, and prevent any possible vision difficulties.

Chapter 4

Reducing the risk of age-related vision loss

As we age, our chance of having age-related vision loss, commonly known as age-related macular degeneration (AMD), grows considerably. AMD is the main cause of vision loss in those over the age of 50, and it may lead to blindness if left untreated. However, there are things that you may do to lower your chance of acquiring AMD and avert blindness.

Eat a nutritious diet: A diet rich in fruits, vegetables, and fatty fish, including salmon and tuna, may help minimize your risk of AMD. These foods include minerals, such as lutein and zeaxanthin, that are vital for maintaining good vision.

Exercise regularly: Exercise has been found to have a protective impact on the eyes, helping to minimize the risk of AMD and other age-related eye disorders.

Wear sunglasses: UV radiation from the sun may damage the retina, increasing your risk of AMD. Wearing sunglasses that filter out UV rays may help protect your eyes from this harm.

Quit smoking: Smoking increases your chance of acquiring AMD and other eye problems, such as cataracts and glaucoma. Quitting smoking may help lessen your risk of certain illnesses.

Get frequent eye examinations: Regular eye exams may assist identify any changes in your vision or possible eye disorders early on, allowing for quick treatment and avoidance of vision loss.

By following these procedures, you may take proactive actions to lower your chance of age-related vision loss and avert blindness.

It is never too late to start taking care of your eyes, so be sure to prioritize your eye health as you age.

Eye disorders and ailments that cause visual loss

There are various eye disorders and ailments that may cause vision loss, including:

Glaucoma: This is a disorder that results in elevated pressure inside the eye, which may damage the optic nerve and cause vision loss. To prevent blindness from glaucoma, it is crucial to have frequent eye examinations and to follow any recommended drugs as instructed.

Cataracts: Cataracts are hazy patches in the lens of the eye that may cause impaired vision. Cataracts may be treated with surgery to remove the hazy lens and replace it with a clear prosthetic lens.

Macular degeneration: This is a disorder that affects the center of the retina, called the macula, which is important for central vision. Macular degeneration may be caused by age, genetics, or other reasons. To prevent or reduce the course of macular degeneration, it is crucial to maintain a balanced diet and avoid smoking.

Diabetic retinopathy: This is a disorder that affects persons with diabetes and leads to damage to the blood vessels of the retina. To prevent blindness from diabetic retinopathy, it is necessary to maintain appropriate blood sugar management and have frequent eye examinations.

Retinal detachment: This is a condition in which the retina gets detached from the underlying tissue of the eye. It may be caused by trauma, genetics, or other reasons. To avoid retinal detachment, it is vital to protect the eyes from damage and to undergo frequent eye checkups.

To avoid vision loss from any of these illnesses, it is crucial to have frequent eye checkups, maintain a healthy lifestyle, and protect the eyes from harm. If you are suffering any signs of vision loss, it is crucial to get medical assistance as soon as possible.

Treatment options for age-related vision loss.

Age-related vision loss, commonly known as age-related macular degeneration (AMD), is a common disorder that affects older persons and may cause considerable vision loss and even blindness. There are various therapy options available for age-related vision loss, and early diagnosis and treatment may help prevent or delay the course of the problem.

Diet and lifestyle changes: Eating a balanced diet rich in fruits, vegetables, and omega-3 fatty acids may help prevent AMD. Quitting smoking and reducing alcohol consumption may also help minimize the chance of getting AMD.

Treatments: Several medications are available to treat AMD, including anti-inflammatory drugs and vitamins that have been demonstrated to delay the course of the illness.

Laser surgery: Laser surgery may be used to eliminate aberrant blood vessels in the eye that might cause vision loss.

Photodynamic therapy: This treatment includes injecting a photosensitizing substance into the bloodstream and then using a specific light to activate the agent and eliminate aberrant blood vessels in the eye.

Implantable micro telescope: This gadget is a small telescope that is implanted in one eye and may aid enhance eyesight by magnifying pictures.

Low vision aids: If vision loss is severe, low vision aids such as magnifiers and special glasses may assist persons with AMD to make the most of their remaining vision.

It is crucial to visit an eye doctor often and to have routine eye examinations to identify any abnormalities in vision early on. Early diagnosis and treatment may help prevent or decrease the course of age-related vision loss and lower the risk of blindness.

Chapter 5

UV radiation and eye health

UV radiation is a form of electromagnetic radiation that is released by the sun and other sources, such as tanning beds. It is categorized into three types: UVA, UVB, and UVC. UVA has the longest wavelength and is the least hazardous, whereas UVC has the shortest wavelength and is the most toxic.

UV radiation is hazardous to the eyes and may cause a range of eye issues, including cataracts, age-related macular degeneration, and skin cancer on the eyelid. It may also cause photokeratitis, a disorder that results in temporary vision loss and pain, and pterygium, a growth on the white area of the eye that can cause visual issues.

To prevent blindness and other eye disorders caused by UV radiation, it is necessary to cover your eyes while you are outside. Here are some tips:

1. Wear sunglasses or eyeglasses with UV protection. Look for glasses that filter 99-100% of UVA and UVB rays.

2. Wear a wide-brimmed hat to shield your face and eyes from the sun's beams.

3. Stay in the shade, particularly during high UV hours (10 am to 4 pm).

4. Wear sunscreen on your face and eyelids to prevent skin cancer.

5. Avoid gazing directly at the sun, since this might cause significant eye damage.

6. Avoid using tanning beds, since they release high quantities of UV radiation that may cause eye issues.

By following these recommendations, you may protect your eyes from the damaging effects of UV radiation and avoid blindness.

Smoking and eye health

Smoking is a substantial risk factor for various eye problems that may lead to blindness. The chemicals in cigarettes may damage the blood vessels in the eye, causing disorders such as age-related macular degeneration (AMD) and diabetic retinopathy. In addition, smoking may also raise the risk of cataracts and glaucoma.

To prevent blindness from smoking, it is vital to stop smoking or never start in the first place. Quitting smoking may help to avoid additional damage to the blood vessels in the eye and may even enhance eyesight in certain circumstances.

In addition to stopping smoking, there are additional measures to safeguard your eye health and avert blindness:

Get frequent eye examinations: Regular eye exams may help to identify any eye issues early on when they are more curable.

Eat a nutritious diet: A diet rich in fruits and vegetables, particularly those strong in antioxidants, may assist to safeguard your eye health.

Wear protective eyewear: Wearing protective eyewear while engaging in activities that may expose your eyes to danger may assist to avoid injury.

Wear sunglasses: Wearing sunglasses may assist to protect your eyes from damaging UV rays, which can lead to the development of cataracts.

Practice excellent hygiene: Proper hygiene, such as washing your hands often and avoiding contacting your eyes with filthy hands, may help to prevent the spread of eye infections.

By following these guidelines, you may assist to safeguard your eye health and avert blindness. Remember that it is never too late to stop smoking and take efforts to enhance your eye health.

High blood pressure and eye health

High blood pressure, also known as hypertension, can have serious consequences for eye health and vision. The high pressure of the blood may damage the blood vessels in the eye, leading to disorders such as glaucoma, retinopathy, and optic nerve damage. These disorders may result in vision loss and perhaps blindness if left unchecked.

To prevent blindness due to high blood pressure, it is vital to maintain healthy blood pressure through lifestyle modifications and medication. This involves eating a balanced diet low in sodium and saturated fats, exercising frequently, and controlling stress. It is also vital to get frequent check-ups with a healthcare practitioner to monitor blood pressure and handle any abnormalities quickly.

If you are already having visual difficulties due to high blood pressure, it is vital to follow the treatment plan given by your healthcare physician. This may involve drugs, lifestyle modifications, and frequent eye examinations. It is also vital to protect your eyes from additional damage by wearing sunglasses and a hat while outdoors, and avoiding activities that may cause eye injuries.

By taking action to control high blood pressure and safeguard your eye health, you may lower your chance of blindness and keep excellent vision for years to come.

Trauma and ocular health

Trauma to the eye may have devastating repercussions and can lead to blindness if not treated swiftly and appropriately. The eye is a fragile and complex organ, and any injury to it may have major repercussions on vision and general eye health.

One of the most frequent causes of eye trauma is physical harm, such as being struck in the eye with an item or getting poked in the eye. This sort of assault may cause substantial damage to the eye, including bleeding, bruising, and swelling. It may also cause damage to the cornea, which is the clear outer layer of the eye that helps protect it from dust, grit, and other debris.

Another prevalent form of ocular damage is chemical injury, which may occur when chemicals come into contact with the eye. This may happen when someone splashes chemicals into their eye or when chemicals from domestic cleaning goods come into contact with the eye. Chemical injury may cause substantial damage to the eye, including burns and scarring, which can lead to vision loss or blindness.

To avoid blindness due to trauma, it is vital to take preventative steps to safeguard the eye. This includes wearing protective eyewear while working with chemicals or in places where there is a danger of eye harm, such as construction sites. It is also vital to seek medical assistance quickly if you experience an eye injury, since timely treatment may help avoid additional damage and preserve eyesight.

In addition to physical and chemical harm, some medical problems may also impact eye health and lead to blindness. For example, illnesses such as diabetes and high blood pressure may cause damage to the blood vessels in the eye, leading to vision loss. To prevent blindness due to these disorders, it is crucial to treat these conditions carefully and follow the instructions of your healthcare expert. This may involve taking drugs, making lifestyle modifications, and obtaining frequent eye checkups.

Overall, it is crucial to take care of your eye health to prevent blindness and other significant eye disorders. This includes safeguarding your eyes from injuries, controlling medical illnesses that might impair eye health, and receiving regular eye examinations to spot any issues early on. By following these steps, you may help protect your eyesight and keep excellent eye health for years to come.

Conclusion

After reading "Preventing blindness," Jack was resolved to do all in his power to prevent blindness. He understood that early identification and treatment were crucial to maintaining sight, so he made sure to obtain frequent check-ups with his eye specialist.

Jack also began adopting more eye-healthy activities into his everyday routine. He made careful to consume a balanced diet rich in vitamins and minerals, particularly those that assist eye health such as lutein and zeaxanthin. He also started wearing sunglasses and a hat anytime he stepped outdoors to shield his eyes from damaging UV radiation.

But Jack didn't stop there. He recognized that many individuals in his town didn't have access to regular eye care, so he launched a program to give free eye tests and spectacles to those in need. He worked with local optometrists and optical establishments to make sure that everyone can see well.

Thanks to Jack's efforts, numerous individuals in his community were able to avert blindness and experience the wonder of sight. He recognized that he had made a meaningful difference in the world and was proud of the influence he had made. And he realized that the information he had learned from "How to avert blindness" had played a vital part in his accomplishment.

In conclusion, blindness is a severe ailment that may have a substantial influence on an individual's quality of life. However, various activities may be done to avoid or lessen the chance of acquiring blindness. These include maintaining excellent general health via a nutritious diet, frequent exercise, and avoiding dangerous behaviors such as smoking and excessive alcohol intake. It is also vital to get regular eye examinations and to safeguard your eyes from harm by wearing suitable protective eyewear while participating in activities such as sports or utilizing hazardous chemicals. By following these rules and receiving prompt medical care for any eye-related issues, it is possible to prevent blindness and retain good eyesight for a lifetime.

Recap of essential points

There are numerous crucial aspects to consider while attempting to prevent blindness:

Maintain excellent eye health: This includes obtaining regular eye examinations, using protective eyewear when appropriate, and avoiding behaviors that may injure your eyes, such as smoking or gazing at screens for extended periods.

Eat a nutritious diet: A diet rich in fruits, vegetables, and nutrients like omega-3 fatty acids will help maintain excellent eye health and lower the chance of vision loss.

Wear sunglasses: Protect your eyes from damaging UV rays by wearing sunglasses while outdoors, particularly during peak hours.

Protect your eyes from injury: Wear protective eyewear while engaging in activities that may represent a danger to your eyes, such as sports or dealing with hazardous chemicals.

Manage chronic conditions: If you have a chronic health condition such as diabetes, high blood pressure, or autoimmune disease, it is crucial to managing it effectively to lower the chance of vision loss.

Follow medication and treatment instructions: If you are given medication or treatment for an eye issue, be sure to follow your doctor's recommendations and attend any follow-up visits.

Educate yourself: Learn about common eye disorders and the signs and symptoms to look for. This will help you spot possible difficulties early and get treatment as required.

www.ingramcontent.com/pod-product-compliance
Lightning Source LLC
Chambersburg PA
CBHW050321220526
45465CB00005B/2076